Pharmacogenomics Basics

Dr. Lusia Fomuso

This book is dedicated to all my children. May your desire to learn new things never fade. I love you all

Pharmacogenomics Basics

Chapter 1: Introduction to Pharmacogenomics

- What is pharmacogenomics?
- Historical Context and Milestones in Pharmacogenomics
- Basic concepts and terminology

Chapter 2: Genetics and Genomics

- What are genes?
- What is DNA?
- What is genomics?

Chapter 3: Drug Metabolism

- How drugs are metabolized in the body
- What is a drug's pharmacokinetics?
- How genetic variation affects drug metabolism

Chapter 4: Types of Genetic Variation and Drug Response

- Single nucleotide polymorphisms (SNPs), Copy number variations (CNVs), Insertions and deletions (indels)
- How genetic variation can affect drug response
- Examples of drugs with known pharmacogenomic effects

Chapter 5: Pharmacogenomic Testing

- What is pharmacogenomic testing?
- How is it done?
- Pros and cons of testing

Chapter 6: Pharmacogenomics in Therapeutic Areas

- Cardiology

Chapter 7: Pharmacogenomics in Therapeutic Areas

- Psychiatry and Neurology

Chapter 8: Pharmacogenomics in Therapeutic Areas

- Oncology

Chapter 9: Pharmacogenomics in Therapeutic Areas

- Gastroenterology and Hepatology

Chapter 10: Ethical and Social Issues

- Ethical considerations in pharmacogenomics
- Social implications of pharmacogenomics

Chapter 11: Current and Future Directions

- Current research in pharmacogenomics
- Potential future applications
- Nutrigenomics

Chapter 12: Resources for Pharmacogenomics and Conclusion

- Websites, organizations, and other resources for learning more about pharmacogenomics
- Summary of key points
- Final comments on the Importance of pharmacogenomics in personalized medicine

Chapter 1: Introduction to Pharmacogenomics

What is pharmacogenomics?

Pharmacogenomics is the study of how an individual's genetic makeup affects their response to medications. It involves analyzing a patient's genetic profile to determine how their body is likely to metabolize a particular drug. This information can be used to personalize treatment plans and choose medications that are most effective for an individual patient, while avoiding drugs that may cause harmful side effects.

Pharmacogenomics combines the fields of pharmacology, the study of how drugs work in the body, and genomics, the study of how genes are inherited and function. The goal of pharmacogenomics is to use genetic information to optimize medication therapy, making it more effective and safer for individual patients. This can help doctors choose the most effective medication and avoid any potential adverse reactions.

The significance of pharmacogenomics lies in its potential to enable personalized medicine and individualized treatment approaches. Traditionally, medications have been prescribed based on a one-size-fits-all approach, if the average patient will respond similarly to a given drug. However, this approach overlooks the inherent genetic differences among individuals, leading to variability in drug response and potentially adverse reactions.

Pharmacogenomics seeks to address this issue by tailoring drug therapy to an individual's genetic profile. By identifying genetic variants associated with drug response, healthcare providers can predict how a patient is likely to metabolize and respond to specific medications. This knowledge allows for the selection of drugs and dosages that are most effective and safe for each patient, minimizing the risk of adverse reactions and increasing treatment efficacy.

The significance of pharmacogenomics in personalized medicine can be seen in various scenarios:

1. Drug Selection: Pharmacogenomic testing can guide the selection of drugs based on an individual's genetic profile. For example, certain genetic variations may affect the response to antidepressant medications, allowing clinicians to choose the most suitable antidepressant for a specific patient.

2. Dose Individualization: Genetic variations can influence how the body metabolizes drugs, affecting their efficacy and toxicity. Pharmacogenomics helps determine optimal drug dosages to achieve the desired therapeutic effect while minimizing adverse effects.

3. Adverse Drug Reactions: Genetic factors play a crucial role in determining an individual's susceptibility to adverse drug reactions. Pharmacogenomic testing can identify patients at higher risk and enable proactive measures to avoid potentially harmful reactions.

4. Precision Cancer Treatment: Pharmacogenomics has particular significance in oncology.

Genetic testing can identify specific gene mutations that drive cancer growth and help tailor targeted therapies to the individual's tumor characteristics, increasing treatment effectiveness and reducing unnecessary side effects. In summary, pharmacogenomics offers the potential to revolutionize medicine by enabling personalized treatment approaches based on an individual's genetic profile. By integrating genetic information into clinical decision-making, healthcare providers can optimize drug therapy, enhance treatment outcomes, and improve patient safety and satisfaction.

Why is pharmacogenomics important?

Pharmacogenomics has the potential to revolutionize the way that medications are prescribed and used. By understanding how a patient's genetic makeup affects their response to medication, doctors can tailor their treatment plans to optimize effectiveness and minimize the risk of side effects.

Some patients may require a higher or lower dose of medication due to their genetic makeup, while others may be at higher risk of adverse reactions. Pharmacogenomics can also help identify which patients are most likely to benefit from a particular medication, which can save time and resources by avoiding trial-and-error approaches to medication therapy.

In addition, pharmacogenomics can help improve drug development by providing insights into how drugs are metabolized, and which patients are most likely to benefit from them.

This can help pharmaceutical companies design more effective and targeted medications. Pharmacogenomics, as a field of study, has a rich historical background marked by key discoveries and milestones. Understanding the historical context helps to appreciate the progress made in pharmacogenomics research and its integration into clinical practice. Here are some notable milestones:

1. Early Observations (1950s-1960s):
    *   The field of pharmacogenomics can be traced back to observations made in the 1950s and 1960s. Researchers noticed individual differences in drug response and adverse reactions, which raised questions about the role of genetics in drug metabolism and efficacy.
2. G6PD Deficiency and Antimalarials (1950s):
    *   One of the earliest examples of pharmacogenomics is the discovery of the association between glucose-6-phosphate dehydrogenase (G6PD) deficiency and adverse reactions to antimalarial drugs like primaquine. This finding highlighted the role of genetic variations in drug response.
3. Thiopurine Methyltransferase (TPMT) and Mercaptopurine (1980s):
    *   In the 1980s, researchers discovered that variations in the TPMT gene influence the metabolism of the anticancer drug mercaptopurine. Individuals with low TPMT activity were found to

be at increased risk of severe toxicity when treated with standard doses of the drug.

4. CYP2D6 and Debrisoquine (1980s):

    - The discovery of the CYP2D6 gene's role in metabolizing the antihypertensive drug debrisoquine marked a significant milestone in pharmacogenomics. Researchers found that certain individuals had reduced CYP2D6 activity, leading to drug accumulation and increased risk of adverse effects.

5. Human Genome Project (1990s):

    - The completion of the Human Genome Project in 2003 was a landmark achievement that provided a comprehensive map of the human genome. This breakthrough laid the foundation for pharmacogenomics research by identifying genetic variations associated with drug response and metabolism.

6. Warfarin and CYP2C9/VKORC1 (2007):

    - The discovery of genetic variants in the CYP2C9 and VKORC1 genes linked to warfarin response revolutionized anticoagulant therapy.
    Understanding an individual's genetic profile for these genes helps predict the optimal dose of warfarin, reducing the risk of bleeding or clotting complications.

7. FDA Guidance on Pharmacogenomics (2005 and ongoing):

    • The U.S. Food and Drug Administration (FDA) has been actively involved in guiding the integration of pharmacogenomics into drug development and clinical practice. The FDA issued its first guidance on pharmacogenomics in 2005, providing recommendations for incorporating genetic information in drug labels.

8. Implementation of Pharmacogenomic Testing (Current Era):

    • In recent years, pharmacogenomic testing has become more accessible and widespread. Several healthcare institutions and clinics have integrated pharmacogenomic testing into their clinical workflows, enabling personalized treatment decisions based on individual genetic profiles.

These milestones highlight the progression of pharmacogenomics from early observations to the current era of personalized medicine. They demonstrate the growing recognition of genetic variations as key factors influencing drug response and the increasing application of pharmacogenomics in clinical practice. The field continues to advance, with ongoing research and discoveries expanding our understanding of the genetic basis of drug response and shaping the future of precision medicine.

Pharmacogenomics involves several key concepts and terms. Some important ones include:

- Genetic variation: Differences in DNA sequence that can affect how genes function. These can include single nucleotide polymorphisms (SNPs), copy number variations (CNVs), and other types of genetic variation.

- Enzymes: Proteins that facilitate chemical reactions in the body. Enzymes are involved in drug metabolism, and genetic variations in enzymes can affect how drugs are metabolized.

- Pharmacokinetics: The study of how drugs are absorbed, distributed, metabolized, and eliminated by the body.

- Pharmacodynamics: The study of how drugs interact with the body to produce their effects.

- Therapeutic index: The ratio of a drug's therapeutic effects to its toxic effects. A higher therapeutic index indicates that a drug is safer and more effective.

- Adverse drug reactions: Harmful or unintended effects of a medication. Adverse drug reactions can be caused by a variety of factors, including genetic variations that affect drug metabolism or sensitivity.

One example of pharmacogenomics in action is the drug Warfarin, which is commonly used as a blood thinner to prevent blood clots. However, Warfarin can have serious side effects, including bleeding, if not properly dosed. In some cases, genetic testing can help determine the most effective dose of Warfarin for a patient, reducing the risk of adverse effects.

Another example is the drug Abacavir, which is used to treat HIV. Some patients have a genetic variation that can cause a severe allergic reaction to the drug. A genetic test can identify patients who are at risk of this reaction, allowing doctors to prescribe an alternative medication.

In another example, the liver enzyme CYP2D6 is responsible for metabolizing many antidepressants and antipsychotics. Some people have genetic variations that result in reduced CYP2D6 activity, leading to slower metabolism of these drugs and potentially higher levels of the drug in the body. This can increase the risk of adverse effects, such as sedation, dizziness, and confusion.

Pharmacogenomics has the potential to revolutionize healthcare by providing more personalized and effective treatments for patients. As our understanding of genetics continues to advance, we can expect to see more applications of pharmacogenomics in clinical practice.

To effectively understand and discuss pharmacogenomics, it is important to become familiar with key terms and concepts in the field. Here are some essential terms and concepts in pharmacogenomics:

1. Genotype: A genotype refers to the genetic makeup of an individual for a specific gene or set of genes. It represents the combination of alleles (alternate forms of a gene) inherited from both parents.

2. Phenotype: Phenotype refers to the observable characteristics or traits of an individual resulting from the interaction between their genotype and the environment. In pharmacogenomics, the phenotype often refers to the individual's response to a drug, including its efficacy and potential side effects.

3. Allele: An allele is one of the alternative forms of a gene located at a specific position (locus) on a chromosome. Everyone inherits two alleles for a given gene, one from each parent.

4. Haplotype: A haplotype is a specific combination of alleles on a single chromosome. Haplotypes can be used to assess the genetic variations within a specific region of the genome.

5. Pharmacogenomic Biomarker: A pharmacogenomic biomarker is a genetic variant or set of variants that is associated with drug response or drug-related traits. These biomarkers can help predict an individual's likelihood of responding to a particular drug, experiencing adverse reactions, or determining optimal dosing.

6. Drug Metabolism: Drug metabolism refers to the biochemical processes by which the body converts drugs into different chemical forms to facilitate their elimination from the body. Genetic variations in drug-metabolizing enzymes can affect the rate at which drugs are metabolized, leading to differences in drug efficacy and toxicity.

7. Pharmacokinetics: Pharmacokinetics refers to the study of how drugs are absorbed, distributed, metabolized, and eliminated by the body. Genetic variations in drug-metabolizing enzymes and drug transporters can influence drug pharmacokinetics, leading to variations in drug concentrations and response.

8. Pharmacodynamics: Pharmacodynamics refers to the study of how drugs interact with their target molecules (e.g., receptors, enzymes) to produce their therapeutic effects. Genetic variations in drug target proteins can affect drug efficacy and response.

9. Therapeutic Index: The therapeutic index is a measure of the safety and efficacy of a drug. It is the ratio between the dose of a drug that produces a therapeutic effect and the dose that produces adverse effects. Pharmacogenomics can help optimize the therapeutic index by selecting drugs and dosages that are most effective and safe for individual patients.

10. Polygenic Variation: Polygenic variation refers to the influence of multiple genetic variants on a particular trait or drug response. Many pharmacogenomic traits are influenced by multiple genes, and understanding polygenic variation helps explain the complexity of drug response variability.

By familiarizing oneself with these key terms and concepts in pharmacogenomics, individuals can better grasp the principles underlying the field and engage in discussions related to personalized medicine, genetic testing, and drug optimization based on an individual's genetic profile.

Chapter 2: Genetics and Genomics

Genetics and genomics are both important fields that play a crucial role in pharmacogenomics. Genetics is the study of how traits are inherited from one generation to another, while genomics is the study of all the genes in an organism's DNA, as well as how they interact with each other and the environment.

Genes

Genes are segments of DNA that provide the instructions for building and maintaining an organism. They control traits such as eye color, height, and susceptibility to certain diseases. Human DNA is made up of about 20,000 to 25,000 genes. Additionally, advances in gene editing and gene therapy may allow for the targeted modification or correction of specific genes that affect drug response. In pharmacogenomics, genes are of particular interest as they can impact how a person responds to medication.

DNA

DNA is central to pharmacogenomics because it contains the genetic information that determines how an individual metabolizes and responds to medications.

As our understanding of genetics and drug response continues to advance, DNA sequencing and analysis are likely to play an increasingly important role in pharmacogenomics. For example, whole-genome sequencing can identify novel genetic variations that may be relevant to medication therapy and lead to the development of new drugs that are tailored to specific genetic profiles. DNA plays a critical role in pharmacogenomics and is likely to be a key focus of research and development in this field in the years to come.

Genomics

Genomics has made tremendous strides in recent years due to advances in technology. Researchers can now sequence an individual's entire genome, which means reading all their DNA base pairs. This allows them to identify genetic variations that may contribute to disease or affect how a person responds to medications.

One of the most important concepts in pharmacogenomics is genetic variation which we will look at in more details in a later chapter. Every person has a unique combination of genetic variations that can influence how their body responds to medication.

These variations can affect how enzymes metabolize drugs in the liver, how proteins interact with drugs in the bloodstream, or how drugs are transported into and out of cells.

Single nucleotide polymorphisms (SNPs) are a type of genetic variation that is particularly important in pharmacogenomics. SNPs are variations in a single nucleotide base pair of DNA that occur in at least 1% of the population. They can affect how genes function and contribute to differences in disease risk and drug response between individuals.

Genetic testing is a tool that can be used to identify genetic variations that may impact medication therapy. There are several types of genetic tests, including genotyping and whole-genome sequencing and these will be covered in a later chapter.

Genotyping tests analyze specific SNPs or genes that are known to be important for drug metabolism or response. Whole-genome sequencing reads all a person's DNA and can identify novel genetic variations that may be relevant to medication therapy.

It's important to note that genetics is not the only factor that influences how a person responds to medication.

Environmental factors such as diet, lifestyle, and exposure to toxins can also play a role. However, understanding a patient's genetic profile can provide important insights into their unique response to medication and help tailor treatment plans for maximum efficacy and safety.

The genetic basis of drug response and variability refers to the influence of genetic variations on an individual's response to medications. Genetic factors play a significant role in how drugs are metabolized, transported, and interact with target proteins in the body. Understanding the genetic basis of drug response can help personalize medication selection, optimize dosing, and reduce the risk of adverse reactions. Here are the key aspects of the genetic basis of drug response and variability:

1. Genetic Variations:
   - Genetic variations are alterations or differences in the DNA sequence of an individual's genome. These variations can occur at the level of a single nucleotide (SNPs), where a single DNA base is replaced, or involve larger segments of DNA, such as copy number variations (CNVs).

   These genetic variations can affect drug response by influencing the function or expression of relevant genes.

2. Pharmacokinetic Genes:
   - Pharmacokinetic genes are involved in the absorption, distribution, metabolism, and elimination of drugs (ADME processes). Variations in these genes can affect drug metabolism, leading to altered drug concentrations in the body.

Examples of pharmacokinetic genes include cytochrome P450 enzymes (e.g., CYP2D6, CYP2C19), drug transporters (e.g., ABCB1, SLCO1B1), and drug-metabolizing enzymes (e.g., TPMT, UGT1A1).

3. Pharmacodynamic Genes:

    - Pharmacodynamic genes are involved in the pharmacological effects of drugs, including drug target proteins, and signaling pathways. Genetic variations in pharmacodynamic genes can influence drug efficacy and response.
      Examples include receptors (e.g., β1-adrenergic receptor), ion channels (e.g., hERG), and enzymes involved in drug action (e.g., COMT).

4. Drug Metabolism:

    - Genetic variations in drug-metabolizing enzymes, such as cytochrome P450 enzymes, can lead to differences in drug metabolism rates. This can result in individuals being categorized as poor metabolizers (PM), intermediate metabolizers (IM), extensive metabolizers (EM), or ultrarapid metabolizers (UM), depending on their genetic variants. These differences in drug metabolism can impact drug efficacy and toxicity.

5. Drug Transport:

- Genetic variations in drug transporters, such as P-glycoprotein (encoded by the ABCB1 gene), can affect the absorption, distribution, and elimination of drugs. Altered drug transporter function can influence drug concentrations in target tissues and affect drug response and toxicity.

6. Pharmacogenomic Biomarkers:

- Pharmacogenomic biomarkers are specific genetic variants that are associated with drug response. These biomarkers can help predict an individual's likelihood of responding to a particular drug or experiencing adverse reactions. Examples include the HLA-B*57:01 allele associated with hypersensitivity to abacavir and the KRAS mutation associated with resistance to certain targeted cancer therapies.

Understanding the genetic basis of drug response and variability allows healthcare providers to make informed decisions regarding drug selection, dosing, and monitoring. Pharmacogenomic testing can identify specific genetic variants relevant to drug response, enabling personalized medicine and improving patient outcomes by maximizing treatment effectiveness and minimizing adverse reactions. By considering an individual's genetic profile, healthcare providers can optimize drug therapy, leading to safer and more effective treatments.

In conclusion, genetics and genomics are fundamental to pharmacogenomics. By understanding how genes interact with medications, doctors and researchers can develop personalized treatment plans that optimize medication therapy and improve patient outcomes. Genetic testing and whole-genome sequencing are valuable tools for identifying genetic variations that may impact medication therapy, but environmental factors must also be taken into consideration in the context of personalized medicine.

Chapter 3: Drug Metabolism

Pharmacokinetics and Pharmacogenomics

Pharmacokinetics is a branch of pharmacology that studies how drugs are absorbed, distributed, metabolized, and eliminated by the body. It encompasses the various processes that a drug undergoes in the body, including its absorption into the bloodstream, distribution to target tissues, metabolism by enzymes, and excretion from the body. The goal of pharmacokinetics is to understand how drugs move through the body to optimize their efficacy and safety.

One important aspect of pharmacokinetics is drug metabolism, which is the process by which the body breaks down a drug into smaller molecules that can be eliminated from the body. Drug metabolism primarily occurs in the liver, where specialized enzymes break down drugs into metabolites. These metabolites are then excreted in the urine or feces.

Genetic variations can impact the function of these enzymes, leading to differences in how individuals metabolize drugs. For instance, some people have genetic variations that result in slow metabolism of drugs, leading to an increased risk of side effects.

Others may have genetic variations that cause them to metabolize drugs more rapidly, leading to a reduced therapeutic effect. Pharmacogenomics is the study of how these genetic variations can affect drug response.

Understanding how genetic variations affect drug metabolism is essential for optimizing medication efficacy and safety. By analyzing a patient's genetic makeup, doctors can tailor medication regimens to optimize the response to the drug while minimizing the risk of adverse effects. For instance, a patient with a genetic variation that causes them to metabolize a drug more slowly may require a lower dose or a different medication altogether.

Pharmacodynamics and Pharmacogenomics

Pharmacodynamics is the study of how drugs interact with the body to produce their effects. It involves understanding the molecular mechanisms by which drugs bind to their targets and modulate their function. By contrast, pharmacokinetics focuses on the absorption, distribution, metabolism, and excretion of drugs in the body.

One of the key factors that influence the pharmacodynamic response to drugs is genetic variation. Genetic variations can affect drug targets, receptors, enzymes, and transporters, which can in turn affect the drug's efficacy and safety. For example, genetic variations in drug targets can alter the affinity of the drug for its target, leading to a change in the drug's potency or efficacy. Similarly, genetic variations in drug metabolizing enzymes can affect the rate and extent of drug metabolism, leading to variations in drug exposure and response.

The field of pharmacogenomics has made significant progress in recent years, with the identification of genetic variants that are associated with variations in drug response. For example, genetic variations in the CYP2C19 gene have been associated with variations in the metabolism of the antiplatelet drug clopidogrel, which is used to prevent blood clots in patients with cardiovascular disease. Patients who have genetic variations that cause them to metabolize clopidogrel more slowly have a higher risk of adverse cardiovascular events, such as heart attack and stroke.

Similarly, genetic variations in the VKORC1 and CYP2C9 genes have been associated with variations in the response to the blood thinner warfarin. Patients who have genetic variations that cause them to metabolize warfarin more slowly require lower doses of the drug to achieve therapeutic anticoagulation.

Pharmacogenomics has important implications for drug development, drug prescribing, and personalized medicine. By understanding how genetic variations affect drug response, researchers can develop drugs that are more effective and safer for specific patient populations. Pharmacogenomics involves the analysis of genetic variation in drug targets, metabolizing enzymes, and transporters, as well as the identification of genetic variants that are associated with variations in drug response.

Clinicians can use genetic testing to identify patients who may be at risk of adverse drug reactions and tailor their medication regimens accordingly. In this way, pharmacogenomics has the potential to improve patient outcomes and reduce healthcare costs. Pharmacogenomics has the potential to reduce adverse drug reactions and improve the effectiveness of medications.

Pharmacokinetics and pharmacogenomics are essential components of personalized medicine. Understanding how drugs are metabolized in the body and how genetic variations can affect drug response is crucial for optimizing medication therapy. Pharmacogenomic testing can provide important insights into a patient's unique drug metabolism, enabling doctors to make more informed treatment decisions.

Chapter 4: Types of Genetic Variation and Drug Response

Genetic variation refers to the differences in DNA sequence between individuals. These variations can have a significant impact on an individual's health, including how they respond to medications. There are several types of genetic variations, including single nucleotide polymorphisms (SNPs), copy number variations (CNVs), and insertions and deletions (indels).

Single nucleotide polymorphisms (SNPs) are the most common type of genetic variation, accounting for about 90% of all human genetic variation. SNPs are single nucleotide changes in DNA that occur when one nucleotide is replaced by another at a specific position in the genome. SNPs can occur in coding or non-coding regions of DNA and can affect gene expression, protein function, and disease susceptibility.

Copy number variations (CNVs) refer to variations in the number of copies of a particular DNA sequence. CNVs can range in size from a few kilobases to several megabases and can occur in coding or non-coding regions of DNA. CNVs can affect gene expression, protein function, and disease susceptibility, and have been linked to a variety of diseases, including autism, schizophrenia, and cancer.

Insertions and deletions (indels) are genetic variations that involve the insertion or deletion of one or more nucleotides in a DNA sequence.

Indels can occur in coding or non-coding regions of DNA and can affect gene expression, protein function, and disease susceptibility. Indels have been linked to a variety of diseases, including cystic fibrosis and Huntington's disease.

Understanding the different types of genetic variation is important in pharmacogenomics, as each type can have a different impact on medication response. For example, some SNPs have been linked to variations in drug metabolism or drug targets, which can affect the efficacy and safety of medications.

Similarly, CNVs and indels can affect gene expression and protein function, which can also impact medication response. The genetic basis of drug response and variability refers to the influence of genetic variations on an individual's response to medications.

Genetic factors play a significant role in how drugs are metabolized, transported, and interact with target proteins in the body. Understanding the genetic basis of drug response can help personalize medication selection, optimize dosing, and reduce the risk of adverse reactions. Here are the key aspects of the genetic basis of drug response and variability:

1. Genetic Variations:
    -   Genetic variations are alterations or differences in the DNA sequence of an individual's genome. These variations can occur at the level of a single nucleotide (SNPs), where a single DNA base is replaced, or involve larger segments of DNA, such as copy number variations (CNVs).

These genetic variations can affect drug response by influencing the function or expression of relevant genes.

2. Pharmacokinetic Genes:

   • Pharmacokinetic genes are involved in the absorption, distribution, metabolism, and elimination of drugs (ADME processes). Variations in these genes can affect drug metabolism, leading to altered drug concentrations in the body. Examples of pharmacokinetic genes include cytochrome P450 enzymes (e.g., CYP2D6, CYP2C19), drug transporters (e.g., ABCB1, SLCO1B1), and drug-metabolizing enzymes (e.g., TPMT, UGT1A1).

3. Pharmacodynamic Genes:

   • Pharmacodynamic genes are involved in the pharmacological effects of drugs, including drug target proteins, and signaling pathways. Genetic variations in pharmacodynamic genes can influence drug efficacy and response. Examples include receptors (e.g., β1-adrenergic receptor), ion channels (e.g., hERG), and enzymes involved in drug action (e.g., COMT).

4. Drug Metabolism:

   • Genetic variations in drug-metabolizing enzymes, such as cytochrome P450 enzymes, can lead to differences in drug metabolism rates.

This can result in individuals being categorized as poor metabolizers (PM), intermediate metabolizers (IM), extensive metabolizers (EM), or ultrarapid metabolizers (UM), depending on their genetic variants. These differences in drug metabolism can impact drug efficacy and toxicity.

5. Drug Transport:

- Genetic variations in drug transporters, such as P-glycoprotein (encoded by the ABCB1 gene), can affect the absorption, distribution, and elimination of drugs. Altered drug transporter function can influence drug concentrations in target tissues and affect drug response and toxicity.

6. Pharmacogenomic Biomarkers:

- Pharmacogenomic biomarkers are specific genetic variants that are associated with drug response. These biomarkers can help predict an individual's likelihood of responding to a particular drug or experiencing adverse reactions.

   Examples include the HLA-B*57:01 allele associated with hypersensitivity to abacavir and the KRAS mutation associated with resistance to certain targeted cancer therapies.

Understanding the genetic basis of drug response and variability allows healthcare providers to make informed decisions regarding drug selection, dosing, and monitoring.

Pharmacogenomic testing can identify specific genetic variants relevant to drug response, enabling personalized medicine and improving patient outcomes by maximizing treatment effectiveness and minimizing adverse reactions. By considering an individual's genetic profile, healthcare providers can optimize drug therapy, leading to safer and more effective treatments.

Drug response to variations

1. Drug transport: Genetic variations can affect how drugs are transported into and out of cells. For example, the drug digoxin is used to treat heart failure, but its efficacy and safety can be influenced by genetic variations in the gene ABCB1, which encodes a protein that transports the drug out of cells. Some people have genetic variations that result in reduced ABCB1 activity, leading to higher levels of digoxin in the body and an increased risk of toxicity.

2. Drug targets: Genetic variations can affect how drugs interact with their target proteins. For example, the drug clopidogrel is used to prevent blood clots in patients with coronary artery disease. However, some patients have genetic variations in the gene CYP2C19, which can result in reduced activation of clopidogrel and a reduced antiplatelet effect. This can increase the risk of heart attack, stroke, or other cardiovascular events.

There are many drugs with known pharmacogenomic effects. The Clinical Pharmacogenetics Implementation Consortium (CPIC) provides guidelines for how to use genetic information to optimize drug therapy. Here are some examples of drugs with known pharmacogenomic effects:

1. Warfarin: Warfarin is a blood thinner used to prevent blood clots. It is metabolized by the enzymes CYP2C9 and VKORC1. Genetic variations in these genes can affect how a patient responds to warfarin. For example, patients with reduced CYP2C9 activity may require lower doses of warfarin, while patients with genetic variations in VKORC1 may require higher doses.

2. Codeine: Codeine is an opioid used to treat pain and cough. It is metabolized by the enzyme CYP2D6 into its active form, morphine. Some people have genetic variations that result in reduced CYP2D6 activity, leading to reduced conversion of codeine to morphine and a reduced analgesic effect.

3. Trastuzumab: Trastuzumab is a monoclonal antibody used to treat breast cancer. It targets the protein HER2, which is overexpressed in some breast cancers. Some patients have genetic variations in the gene HER2, which can affect their response to trastuzumab. For example, patients with HER2 amplification may have a better response to trastuzumab than patients without HER2 amplification.

In conclusion, genetic variation can affect how drugs are metabolized, transported, and interact with their target proteins, which can influence their efficacy and safety. Understanding how genetic variation affects drug response is an important part of pharmacogenomics and can help tailor drug therapy to optimize patient outcomes.

Chapter 5: Pharmacogenomics Testing

Genotyping and sequencing are fundamental laboratory techniques used in pharmacogenomics to identify genetic variations that influence drug response. These techniques allow researchers and clinicians to analyze an individual's genetic profile and determine the presence of specific genetic markers associated with drug metabolism, drug targets, and treatment outcomes. Here are some common laboratory techniques used in genotyping and sequencing for pharmacogenomics:

1. Polymerase Chain Reaction (PCR):

    - PCR is a widely used technique in molecular biology and pharmacogenomics. It allows for the amplification of specific regions of DNA, making it possible to detect genetic variations in target genes. PCR involves cycles of DNA denaturation, primer annealing, and DNA synthesis using a DNA polymerase enzyme. PCR can be used to amplify specific regions of interest before genotyping or sequencing.

2. Sanger Sequencing:

    - Sanger sequencing, also known as chain termination sequencing, is a classic DNA sequencing method. It involves DNA amplification by PCR, followed by incorporation of chain-terminating nucleotides during DNA synthesis.

The resulting fragments are separated by size using gel electrophoresis, and the DNA sequence is determined based on the order of terminated fragments. Sanger sequencing is suitable for analyzing individual genes or specific genomic regions.

3. Next-Generation Sequencing (NGS):

- NGS technologies have revolutionized genomic research and pharmacogenomics by enabling high-throughput sequencing of DNA. NGS allows for the simultaneous sequencing of millions of DNA fragments, providing comprehensive genetic information. Different NGS platforms, such as Illumina, Ion Torrent, and PacBio, offer various sequencing approaches and applications. NGS can be used to sequence entire genomes, exomes (protein-coding regions), targeted gene panels, or RNA (transcriptome) for pharmacogenomic studies.

4. Microarray Genotyping:

- Microarray technology uses a grid of DNA probes to detect specific genetic variants across the genome. The DNA samples are hybridized to the microarray, and the fluorescence intensity is measured to determine the presence or absence of specific genetic markers. Microarray genotyping can analyze many genetic variants simultaneously, making it efficient for pharmacogenomic studies that focus on predefined genetic markers.

5. Mass Spectrometry:

- Mass spectrometry-based genotyping methods utilize the principles of mass spectrometry to identify and quantify specific genetic variations.

  Techniques such as matrix-assisted laser desorption/ionization time-of-flight (MALDI-TOF) and selected reaction monitoring (SRM) allow for the high-throughput analysis of genetic variants. Mass spectrometry-based genotyping is often used for single nucleotide polymorphism (SNP) genotyping and detection of specific genetic variations.

6. Digital PCR:

- Digital PCR is a sensitive technique used for absolute quantification of DNA molecules. It partitions a DNA sample into thousands of individual reactions, allowing the detection and counting of specific genetic variants. Digital PCR is particularly useful for detecting rare genetic variants and accurately determining their abundance in a sample.

7. DNA Microarrays for Gene Expression Analysis:

- Gene expression microarrays measure the levels of gene expression for thousands of genes simultaneously.

They allow researchers to study how genetic variations influence gene expression patterns and identify biomarkers associated with drug response. Gene expression microarrays can help uncover gene expression signatures relevant to pharmacogenomics and personalized medicine.

These laboratory techniques enable researchers and healthcare professionals to identify and analyze genetic variations relevant to drug response. They provide valuable information for individualizing drug therapy and making informed treatment decisions based on an individual's genetic profile. The choice of technique depends on the specific research or clinical question, the number of genetic markers of interest, and the available resources and infrastructure.

Bioinformatics plays a crucial role in analyzing the large volumes of data generated in pharmacogenomics research. It involves the use of computational tools, algorithms, and databases to process, interpret, and extract meaningful information from genomic and pharmacogenomic data. Here are some commonly used bioinformatics tools for analyzing pharmacogenomic data:

1. Alignment and Variant Calling Tools:

   - Alignment tools, such as Bowtie, BWA, and STAR, are used to map DNA sequencing reads to a reference genome. They align the short reads generated by sequencing platforms to the appropriate genomic location.

Variant calling tools, such as GATK (Genome Analysis Toolkit), SAMtools, and FreeBayes, identify genetic variants, such as single nucleotide polymorphisms (SNPs), insertions, deletions, and structural variations, by comparing the aligned reads to the reference genome.

2. Database Resources:

   • Databases provide a wealth of curated genomic and pharmacogenomic data that can be used for variant annotation, interpretation, and association studies. Resources like dbSNP, ClinVar, PharmGKB, and COSMIC contain information on genetic variants, their frequencies, functional annotations, and their associations with drug response or disease.

3. Variant Annotation Tools:

   • Variant annotation tools, such as ANNOVAR, SnpEff, and VEP (Variant Effect Predictor), annotate genetic variants based on their functional impact. They provide information on the potential effects of variants on protein structure, gene function, regulatory elements, and known functional domains. Annotation tools help prioritize variants for further analysis and interpretation.

4. Pathway Analysis Tools:

   • Pathway analysis tools, such as Ingenuity Pathway Analysis (IPA), Gene Set Enrichment Analysis (GSEA), and Reactome, enable the identification of biological pathways, gene networks, and molecular interactions associated with drug response or specific phenotypes. These tools help uncover underlying mechanisms and provide insights into the biological processes influenced by genetic variants.

5. Pharmacogenomic Prediction Tools:

    - Pharmacogenomic prediction tools, such as PMKB (Precision Medicine Knowledgebase), CPIC (Clinical Pharmacogenetics Implementation Consortium), and PreCise-PGx, offer evidence-based guidelines and recommendations for drug dosing and treatment selection based on an individual's genetic profile. These tools integrate pharmacogenomic data, clinical evidence, and drug-specific information to guide therapeutic decisions.

6. Statistical Analysis Tools:

    - Statistical analysis tools, such as PLINK, R, and SAS, enable the identification of genetic associations with drug response or disease outcomes. They facilitate genotype-phenotype correlation analysis, population stratification assessment, and statistical modeling to identify genetic markers associated with drug efficacy, toxicity, or treatment outcomes.

7. Data Visualization Tools:

- Data visualization tools, such as the Integrative Genomics Viewer (IGV), UCSC Genome Browser, and R packages (e.g., ggplot2), provide graphical representation of genomic and pharmacogenomic data. Visualization tools help researchers and clinicians interpret complex data sets, explore genetic variants, and identify patterns or trends.

These bioinformatics tools, among others, aid in the analysis, interpretation, and translation of pharmacogenomic data into actionable insights. They enable researchers and healthcare professionals to identify clinically relevant genetic markers, understand their functional implications, and apply this knowledge to personalize drug therapy and improve patient outcomes. It is important to select the appropriate tools based on the specific analysis requirements, data type, and available computational resources.

Pharmacogenomics testing is a type of genetic testing that involves analyzing a patient's DNA to identify genetic variations that may affect their response to medications.

Here is a general process for pharmacogenomic testing:

1. Sample collection: A sample of the patient's DNA is collected, typically through a blood draw, cheek swab, or saliva sample.

2. DNA isolation: The DNA is extracted from the sample using various methods, such as column purification or magnetic bead separation.

3. Genetic analysis: The DNA is then analyzed using various techniques, including genotyping or whole-genome sequencing, to identify genetic variations that may affect drug response. Genotyping tests analyze specific genetic variations that are known to be important for drug metabolism or response, while whole-genome sequencing reads all a person's DNA and can identify novel genetic variations that may be relevant to medication therapy.

4. Data interpretation: Once the genetic analysis is complete, the results must be interpreted in the context of the patient's medical history and current medication regimen. This can be a complex process, as there are many genetic variations that can potentially affect drug response and not all of them have been well-studied.

5. Clinical application: Based on the results of the genetic analysis and data interpretation, the healthcare provider can make recommendations for adjusting medication therapy to optimize efficacy and minimize the risk of adverse drug reactions.

There are several companies that offer pharmacogenomic testing and these companies typically provide test kits that can be ordered by a healthcare provider and performed at a home and then mailed to a laboratory. In some cases, insurance may cover the cost of the test, although this varies depending on the specific test and the patient's insurance plan.

It's important to note that pharmacogenomic testing is still an emerging field and there are many challenges to implementing it in clinical practice. These challenges include the need for standardized testing methods and interpretation guidelines, as well as addressing issues related to data privacy and discrimination. However, as more research is conducted and more drugs are developed with known pharmacogenomic effects, testing is likely to become an increasingly important tool for optimizing medication therapy and improving patient outcomes.

Pharmacogenomic testing can also be used to identify patients who may benefit from certain medications, such as those with certain genetic variations associated with increased response to certain antidepressants or cancer treatments. Pharmacogenomic testing has shown promising results in improving medication therapy by tailoring treatment to a patient's unique genetic profile. For example, the FDA has issued several labeling changes for medications based on pharmacogenomic testing results, including clopidogrel, codeine, and abacavir.

Clopidogrel, an antiplatelet medication used to prevent heart attacks and strokes, is activated by the liver enzyme CYP2C19. Patients who have reduced function of this enzyme due to genetic variations may have a decreased response to the drug, which can increase the risk of adverse cardiovascular events. As a result, the FDA recommends that patients who are going to receive clopidogrel undergo genetic testing for CYP2C19 variants.

Codeine is a pain reliever that is metabolized by the liver enzyme CYP2D6 into its active form, morphine. Patients who have reduced function of this enzyme due to genetic variations may experience reduced pain relief or even toxicity from codeine. The FDA has issued a warning about the use of codeine in children who have certain genetic variations of CYP2D6 and recommends considering alternative pain medications.

Abacavir which we mentioned earlier is an antiretroviral medication used to treat HIV. A small percentage of patients who take abacavir develop a hypersensitivity reaction that can be life-threatening. This reaction is strongly associated with the presence of a specific genetic variation, HLA-B*57:01. The FDA recommends genetic testing for this variant before starting abacavir therapy.

As mentioned, the interpretation of test results can be complex and challenging, and not all genetic variations that can potentially affect drug response have been well-studied. Additionally, the cost of testing may not be covered by insurance, which can limit access for some patients.

In summary, pharmacogenomic testing has the potential to improve medication therapy by tailoring treatment to a patient's unique genetic profile. As more research is conducted and more drugs are developed with known pharmacogenomic effects, testing is likely to become even more important for optimizing medication therapy and improving patient outcomes.

Chapter 6: Pharmacogenomics in Cardiology

Genetic variants can significantly influence an individual's response to cardiovascular drugs, including antiplatelet agents, statins, and beta-blockers. Understanding these genetic factors is crucial for optimizing treatment outcomes and tailoring medication regimens. Here are some examples of genetic variants that affect response to commonly used cardiovascular drugs:

1. Antiplatelet Agents:

   Clopidogrel: The CYP2C19 gene plays a vital role in the activation of clopidogrel, an antiplatelet agent commonly used after stent placement or in the management of acute coronary syndromes. Genetic variations in CYP2C19 can lead to reduced drug activation and decreased antiplatelet effect, resulting in an increased risk of adverse cardiovascular events. Testing for CYP2C19 variants helps identify patients who may require alternative antiplatelet therapy or adjusted dosing.

2. Statins:

   SLCO1B1: The SLCO1B1 gene encodes the organic anion-transporting polypeptide 1B1, which is responsible for the hepatic uptake of statins such as simvastatin and pravastatin. Variations in SLCO1B1 have been associated with altered statin pharmacokinetics, leading to differences in drug efficacy and the risk of statin-induced myopathy. Genetic testing for SLCO1B1 variants can help guide statin selection and dosing adjustments.

3. Beta-Blockers:

   ADRB1 and ADRB2: The ADRB1 and ADRB2 genes encode beta-1 and beta-2 adrenergic receptors, respectively, which are targeted by beta-blockers. Genetic variations in these genes can impact the response to beta-blockers in conditions such as hypertension, heart failure, and arrhythmias. For example, certain ADRB1 gene variants have been associated with reduced response to beta-blockers in heart failure patients. Genetic testing for ADRB1 and ADRB2 variants can assist in selecting the most appropriate beta-blocker or alternative treatment options.

   It is important to note that these are just a few examples, and there are numerous other genetic variants that can influence the response to cardiovascular drugs. Pharmacogenomic testing can help identify these variants and guide treatment decisions, allowing for personalized medication regimens that optimize efficacy and minimize adverse effects. Integrating pharmacogenomics into cardiovascular care has the potential to improve treatment outcomes and enhance patient safety.

Impact of pharmacogenomics on individualized antiplatelet therapy for cardiovascular diseases

Pharmacogenomics plays a significant role in individualizing antiplatelet therapy for cardiovascular diseases. By analyzing specific genetic markers, clinicians can identify patients who are more likely to respond to certain antiplatelet agents and those who may be at an increased risk of adverse events.

Here's an overview of the impact of pharmacogenomics on individualized antiplatelet therapy:

1. Clopidogrel and CYP2C19 Genotype:
   - Clopidogrel is a commonly prescribed antiplatelet agent used in the management of acute coronary syndromes and after stent placement. The CYP2C19 gene encodes the enzyme responsible for converting clopidogrel into its active form. Genetic variations in CYP2C19 can result in reduced enzyme activity, leading to decreased effectiveness of clopidogrel.
   - Pharmacogenomic testing for CYP2C19 genotype helps identify patients who are poor metabolizers of clopidogrel. Poor metabolizers have a higher risk of adverse cardiovascular events, such as stent thrombosis or myocardial infarction. Based on the genotype, alternative antiplatelet agents, such as prasugrel or ticagrelor, may be recommended for patients with reduced clopidogrel metabolism.

2. Prasugrel and CYP2C19 Genotype:
   - Prasugrel is another antiplatelet agent used in the management of acute coronary syndromes and after stent placement. Like clopidogrel, prasugrel requires activation by CYP2C19. However,

the impact of CYP2C19 genotype on prasugrel response is less pronounced than with clopidogrel.

- Genetic testing for CYP2C19 genotype may still be considered in cases where there is uncertainty about the optimal antiplatelet therapy. However, routine testing for CYP2C19 genotype is not typically required before initiating prasugrel.

3. Ticagrelor and Genetic Variants:

- Ticagrelor is an oral antiplatelet agent that does not require activation by CYP2C19. Genetic variations in other genes, such as ABCB1 and SLCO1B1, have been studied for their impact on ticagrelor response.

- Although genetic testing for ticagrelor response is not routinely recommended, ongoing research is investigating the potential role of these genetic variants in guiding ticagrelor therapy.

4. Genetic Testing in Dual Antiplatelet Therapy (DAPT):

- Dual antiplatelet therapy (DAPT) with aspirin and an additional antiplatelet agent, such as clopidogrel, prasugrel, or ticagrelor, is often prescribed following percutaneous coronary intervention or in the setting of acute coronary syndromes.

- Pharmacogenomic testing can help identify patients who are at increased risk of adverse events or treatment failure with specific antiplatelet agents. This information can guide the selection of the most appropriate antiplatelet therapy and individualize DAPT regimens.

By incorporating pharmacogenomic testing into clinical practice, healthcare providers can personalize antiplatelet therapy for cardiovascular diseases, improving treatment outcomes and reducing the risk of adverse events. It allows for a more targeted approach to antiplatelet drug selection, ensuring that patients receive the most effective and safe treatment based on their genetic profile.

Considerations for pharmacogenomic testing in the treatment of hypertension and heart failure

Pharmacogenomic testing can play a valuable role in the treatment of hypertension and heart failure by providing insights into a patient's genetic makeup and how it may influence their response to certain medications. Here are some key considerations for pharmacogenomic testing in the context of these conditions:

1. Drug selection: Pharmacogenomic testing can help identify genetic variations that may affect an individual's response to specific antihypertensive and heart failure medications. By analyzing a patient's genetic profile, clinicians can better predict their likelihood of benefiting from certain drugs or experiencing adverse effects. This information can guide drug selection and dosage adjustments to optimize treatment outcomes.

2. Individualized dosing: Genetic variations can impact drug metabolism, efficacy, and toxicity. Pharmacogenomic testing can identify specific genetic markers associated with altered drug metabolism enzymes, such as cytochrome P450 enzymes, which play a crucial role in metabolizing many medications. This information can guide individualized dosing strategies to achieve optimal therapeutic levels while minimizing the risk of side effects.

3. Adverse drug reactions: Certain antihypertensive and heart failure medications may have a higher risk of adverse drug reactions in patients with specific genetic variants. Pharmacogenomic testing can identify these variants and help clinicians avoid prescribing medications that may pose a higher risk of adverse events, such as severe hypotension or drug-induced cardiotoxicity.

4. Treatment response prediction: Genetic variations can influence an individual's response to medications. Pharmacogenomic testing can provide insights into the likelihood of treatment response and guide clinicians in selecting the most appropriate medication or combination therapy. For example, in hypertension, some genetic markers may suggest a better response to diuretics, ACE inhibitors, or calcium channel blockers, while others may indicate a preference for beta-blockers or angiotensin receptor blockers.

5. Treatment cost-effectiveness: Pharmacogenomic testing can potentially contribute to cost-effective treatment strategies. By identifying genetic

markers associated with treatment response or adverse events, clinicians can avoid prescribing medications that are less likely to be effective or more likely to cause harm. This approach may help optimize medication choices, minimize trial-and-error prescribing, and reduce unnecessary healthcare costs.

6. Patient counseling and adherence: Pharmacogenomic testing can enhance patient education and counseling. By explaining how genetic factors influence medication response, clinicians can empower patients to make informed decisions about their treatment. Understanding their genetic profile may also motivate patients to adhere to prescribed medications, knowing that the chosen drugs are more likely to be effective and well-tolerated based on their genetic information.

It's important to note that while pharmacogenomic testing has the potential to enhance treatment outcomes, it should be used as a complementary tool alongside clinical judgment and standard diagnostic practices. The interpretation of genetic results requires expertise, and the field of pharmacogenomics is continuously evolving. Therefore, collaboration between clinicians and genetic specialists is crucial to ensure appropriate utilization and interpretation of pharmacogenomic testing in the context of hypertension and heart failure treatment.

Here are a few case studies that illustrate the application of pharmacogenomics in cardiovascular medicine:

1. Warfarin and VKORC1/CYP2C9 Genotyping: Warfarin is an anticoagulant commonly used to prevent blood clots in cardiovascular conditions. However, its optimal dosage can vary greatly among individuals due to genetic factors. Genotyping of the VKORC1 and CYP2C9 genes can provide valuable information about an individual's response to warfarin. For example, a study published in Circulation in 2009 examined the impact of genotype-guided warfarin dosing on clinical outcomes. The study found that patients who received genetically guided dosing had a significantly reduced risk of bleeding and thromboembolic events compared to those receiving standard dosing.

2. Clopidogrel and CYP2C19 Genotyping: Clopidogrel is an antiplatelet medication used in the treatment of cardiovascular diseases, such as acute coronary syndromes and after stent placement. However, some individuals have genetic variations in the CYP2C19 gene that affect clopidogrel's activation. Genotyping for CYP2C19 can help identify poor metabolizers who may have reduced drug efficacy and an increased risk of cardiovascular events. A study published in the New England Journal of Medicine in 2010 demonstrated that CYP2C19 genotyping could identify patients at higher risk for adverse cardiovascular outcomes, leading to a potential modification of treatment strategies, such as alternative antiplatelet therapies.

3. Beta-Blockers and ADRB1 Genotyping: Beta-blockers are commonly used in the management of hypertension and heart failure. The ADRB1 gene encodes the β1-adrenergic receptor, which is the target for beta-blockers. Genetic variations in ADRB1 can influence an individual's response to beta-blocker therapy. A study published in the Journal of the American College of Cardiology in 2013 investigated the impact of ADRB1 genotype on outcomes in heart failure patients receiving beta-blockers. The study found that certain ADRB1 genotypes were associated with a greater reduction in heart failure-related hospitalizations and mortality when patients were treated with beta-blockers.

These case studies highlight how pharmacogenomic testing can provide valuable insights into individual drug responses and guide personalized treatment decisions in cardiovascular medicine. By considering genetic variations that impact drug metabolism, efficacy, and adverse events, clinicians can optimize medication selection, dosing, and treatment strategies to improve patient outcomes. However, it's important to note that these case studies represent specific scenarios, and pharmacogenomic testing recommendations may vary based on factors such as clinical guidelines, patient characteristics, and availability of testing resources.

Chapter 7: Pharmacogenomics in Psychiatry and Neurology

Genetic factors can significantly influence the response and adverse effects of psychotropic medications, including antidepressants and antipsychotics. Here are some key genetic considerations:

1. Antidepressants: a. CYP2D6 Genotype: The CYP2D6 gene encodes an enzyme responsible for metabolizing many antidepressants, including selective serotonin reuptake inhibitors (SSRIs) and tricyclic antidepressants. Genetic variations in CYP2D6 can lead to differences in drug metabolism and plasma concentrations. Poor metabolizers may experience reduced drug efficacy, while ultrarapid metabolizers may be at higher risk of adverse effects or require lower dosages. b. SLC6A4 Genotype: The SLC6A4 gene influences the serotonin transporter, which is the target of SSRIs. Variations in this gene, such as the serotonin transporter-linked polymorphic region (5-HTTLPR), have been associated with differential treatment response and susceptibility to adverse effects.

   c. HTR2A Genotype: Genetic variations in the HTR2A gene, which encodes the serotonin 2A receptor, have been linked to antidepressant response. Some studies suggest that certain variations may predict a better response to specific classes of antidepressants, such as SSRIs or serotonin-norepinephrine reuptake inhibitors (SNRIs).

2. Antipsychotics: a. CYP2D6 and CYP2C19 Genotypes: Like antidepressants, the metabolism of many antipsychotics, such as risperidone and haloperidol, is influenced by CYP2D6 and CYP2C19 enzymes. Genetic variations in these genes can affect drug metabolism and plasma concentrations, leading to variable treatment response and risk of adverse effects. b. DRD2 Genotype: The dopamine D2 receptor, encoded by the DRD2 gene, is the target of many antipsychotics. Genetic variations in DRD2 have been associated with treatment response and side effect profiles. For example, certain polymorphisms may contribute to increased susceptibility to extrapyramidal symptoms (EPS) or hyperprolactinemia.

c. HTR2C Genotype: The serotonin 2C receptor, encoded by the HTR2C gene, is involved in the mechanism of action of some antipsychotics. Genetic variations in HTR2C have been linked to treatment response and the risk of side effects, including weight gain and metabolic disturbances.

It's important to note that while these genetic factors can provide valuable insights, they are just one piece of the puzzle in determining the most appropriate psychotropic medication and dosage for an individual. Clinical factors, patient history, and therapeutic monitoring should also be considered when making treatment decisions. Pharmacogenomic testing can assist clinicians in personalized prescribing and optimizing treatment outcomes, but it should be integrated with comprehensive clinical assessments and ongoing monitoring of patients' responses to medication.

Pharmacogenomic testing for optimizing psychiatric medication selection and dosing

Pharmacogenomic testing can be a valuable tool for optimizing psychiatric medication selection and dosing.

By analyzing an individual's genetic makeup, clinicians can gain insights into how their genetic variations may influence the metabolism, efficacy, and adverse effects of psychiatric medications. Here are some key considerations for pharmacogenomic testing in the context of optimizing psychiatric medication:

1. Antidepressants:

    - Drug metabolism enzymes: Genetic variations in genes encoding drug-metabolizing enzymes, such as CYP2D6 and CYP2C19, can impact the metabolism of antidepressants. This information helps identify individuals who may be poor metabolizers or ultrarapid metabolizers, guiding appropriate dosage adjustments.

    - Serotonin transporter: Genetic variants in the SLC6A4 gene, which encodes the serotonin transporter protein, have been associated with differential response and adverse effects to SSRIs. Testing for these variants can inform the choice of SSRIs or alternative treatment options.

- Other relevant genes: Genes such as HTR2A and FKBP5 have been implicated in antidepressant response. Pharmacogenomic testing can provide information about variations in these genes, which may help guide treatment decisions.

2. Antipsychotics:

- Drug metabolism enzymes: Genetic variations in CYP2D6 and CYP2C19 can impact the metabolism of antipsychotics, such as risperidone and haloperidol. Testing for these variations can inform dosage adjustments and help predict individual responses.

- Dopamine receptors: Genetic variants in genes encoding dopamine receptors, such as DRD2, can influence antipsychotic response and the risk of side effects. Pharmacogenomic testing can identify these variants and guide the choice of antipsychotics or dosing strategies.

- Other relevant genes: Genes like HTR2C and COMT have been associated with antipsychotic response and side effects. Testing for variations in these genes can provide additional insights for optimizing treatment outcomes.

3. Anxiolytics and Mood Stabilizers:

- Drug metabolism enzymes: Genetic variations in drug-metabolizing enzymes, including CYP2C19 and CYP2D6, can impact the metabolism of anxiolytics (e.g., benzodiazepines) and mood stabilizers (e.g., lithium).

Pharmacogenomic testing can inform dosage adjustments and help tailor treatment regimens.

- GABA receptors and other relevant genes: Genetic variants in genes involved in the GABAergic system and other neurotransmitter systems, such as GABRA2 and GAD1, may influence the response and adverse effects of anxiolytics and mood stabilizers. Testing for these variants can provide additional guidance for medication selection.

Pharmacogenomic testing can enhance personalized treatment approaches, reduce trial-and-error prescribing, and potentially improve treatment outcomes in psychiatry. However, it's important to note that pharmacogenomic testing should be used as a complementary tool alongside clinical judgment and ongoing patient monitoring.

The interpretation of genetic results requires expertise, and the field of pharmacogenomics is continuously evolving. Therefore, collaboration between clinicians, genetic specialists, and appropriate counseling support is crucial to ensure the effective integration of pharmacogenomic information into psychiatric medication management.

Pharmacogenomics has the potential to play a significant role in the treatment of neurodegenerative disorders, such as Alzheimer's disease and Parkinson's disease. Here are some key considerations for the application of pharmacogenomics in these conditions:

1. Alzheimer's Disease:

   - Apolipoprotein E (APOE) Genotype: The APOE gene is a well-established genetic risk factor for late-onset Alzheimer's disease. The APOE ε4 allele is associated with an increased risk of developing the disease. Pharmacogenomic testing can help identify individuals with this high-risk genotype and enable early interventions, including lifestyle modifications and potential participation in clinical trials targeting APOE-related pathways.

   - Cholinesterase Inhibitors: Cholinesterase inhibitors, such as donepezil, rivastigmine, and galantamine, are commonly prescribed for symptomatic treatment of Alzheimer's disease. Genetic variations in genes encoding drug-metabolizing enzymes, such as CYP2D6 and CYP3A4, can influence the metabolism and response to these medications. Pharmacogenomic testing can guide dosage adjustments and personalized treatment decisions.

   - Drug Targets and Pathways: Genetic variations in genes involved in the processing and clearance of amyloid beta, such as APP and PSEN1/2, may impact disease progression and treatment response. Pharmacogenomics research is exploring the potential for targeting specific genetic variants and pathways to develop precision therapies for Alzheimer's disease.

2. Parkinson's Disease:

- L-DOPA and Dopamine Agonists: L-DOPA, the primary medication for Parkinson's disease, and dopamine agonists, such as pramipexole and ropinirole, are commonly used to manage motor symptoms. Genetic variations in genes like COMT and DRD2 can influence the response to these medications and the risk of motor complications. Pharmacogenomic testing can inform personalized dosing and treatment strategies.

- Monoamine Oxidase B (MAO-B) Inhibitors: MAO-B inhibitors, such as selegiline and rasagiline, are used as adjunctive therapy in Parkinson's disease. Genetic variations in the gene encoding MAO-B, MAOB, may impact the metabolism and response to these inhibitors. Pharmacogenomic testing can help guide dosage adjustments and treatment decisions.

- Other Genetic Factors: Multiple genes associated with Parkinson's disease, including SNCA, LRRK2, and PARKIN, have been identified. Pharmacogenomics research is exploring the potential impact of these genetic variations on disease progression, treatment response, and the development of targeted therapies.

It's important to note that while pharmacogenomic testing holds promise, its utility in neurodegenerative disorders is still being actively researched and refined. The complexity of these conditions, with multiple genetic and environmental factors at play, necessitates a comprehensive approach that combines genetic information with clinical assessment and monitoring.

Additionally, genetic testing may have implications for family members and ethical considerations should be considered. Collaboration between neurologists, genetic specialists, and other healthcare providers is crucial to ensure the appropriate integration of pharmacogenomic information into the management of neurodegenerative disorders.

Here are a few case studies that demonstrate the role of pharmacogenomics in psychiatry and neurology:

1. Case Study: Pharmacogenomic Testing in Antidepressant Selection: In a study published in The American Journal of Psychiatry in 2013, 1,167 patients with major depressive disorder were randomized to receive either treatment-as-usual or treatment guided by a pharmacogenomic test panel. The panel included genetic variations in genes involved in drug metabolism and response to antidepressants. The study found that patients who received guided treatment had a significantly higher response rate and remission rate compared to those receiving treatment-as-usual. The findings suggested that pharmacogenomic testing can aid in the selection of antidepressants and improve treatment outcomes.

2. Case Study: Genetic Testing for Warfarin Dosing in Psychiatry: A case study published in the Journal of Clinical Psychopharmacology in 2011 highlighted the role of pharmacogenomic testing in guiding warfarin dosing in a patient with schizophrenia and comorbid anxiety disorder. The patient had a history of subtherapeutic and supratherapeutic INR (international normalized ratio) values while on warfarin therapy. Genetic testing for CYP2C9 and VKORC1 variants helped identify the patient's poor metabolizer status and guided dosage adjustments, resulting in improved INR stability and reduced bleeding risk.

3. Case Study: Pharmacogenomics in Antipsychotic Medication Selection: In a case report published in Psychiatric Services in 2016, a patient with treatment-resistant schizophrenia underwent pharmacogenomic testing to guide antipsychotic medication selection. The patient had previously experienced inadequate response and side effects with multiple antipsychotics.

Genetic testing revealed a CYP2D6 ultra-rapid metabolizer status, which explained the rapid clearance of some antipsychotics. Based on the results, the patient's treatment was modified to utilize antipsychotics that were not primarily metabolized by CYP2D6. The patient showed a substantial improvement in symptom control and tolerability.

4. Case Study: Pharmacogenomics in Parkinson's Disease Treatment: A case report published in Clinical Neuropharmacology in 2018 described a patient with Parkinson's disease who experienced motor complications, such as dyskinesias, despite optimized treatment with levodopa. Pharmacogenomic testing was performed to identify genetic variants in the COMT gene. The patient was found to be a poor metabolizer due to a specific COMT variant, resulting in elevated levodopa metabolism. Based on the results, the patient's treatment was modified by reducing the levodopa dosage and adding a COMT inhibitor, resulting in a reduction of dyskinesias and improved motor control.

These case studies demonstrate how pharmacogenomic testing can provide valuable insights into medication selection, dosing adjustments, and treatment response in psychiatry and neurology. By considering an individual's genetic variations, clinicians can personalize treatment strategies, improve medication efficacy, and minimize the risk of adverse effects. However, it's important to note that these case studies represent specific scenarios, and pharmacogenomic testing recommendations may vary based on individual patient characteristics, clinical guidelines, and available testing resources.

Chapter 8: Pharmacogenomics in Oncology

Pharmacogenomics has significant potential in the field of oncology, where personalized treatment plans can be developed based on a patient's individual genetic makeup. By identifying specific genetic mutations or biomarkers, oncologists can choose the most effective treatments for individual patients, minimizing adverse effects and maximizing therapeutic efficacy.

The field of pharmacogenomics in oncology aims to identify genetic markers that can predict a patient's response to cancer treatments, allowing for personalized and more effective therapy. Here is an overview of pharmacogenomics in oncology and its impact on personalized cancer treatment:

1. Genetic Variations and Drug Response:

    *   Genetic variations in cancer-related genes can significantly impact an individual's response to cancer treatments. These variations can affect drug metabolism, drug targets, DNA repair mechanisms, and signaling pathways involved in cancer growth and progression. Pharmacogenomic studies aim to identify specific genetic markers associated with drug efficacy, toxicity, and overall treatment outcomes.

2. Personalized Treatment Selection:

    *   Pharmacogenomic testing allows oncologists to personalize treatment selection based on an individual's genetic profile.

By analyzing specific genetic markers, such as mutations, gene amplifications, or gene expression patterns, clinicians can identify the most suitable treatment options for each patient. This approach helps avoid ineffective treatments and minimizes unnecessary toxicity.

3. Predicting Drug Efficacy:
   - Pharmacogenomic markers can help predict a patient's response to specific cancer drugs. For example, in breast cancer, the presence of HER2 gene amplification or overexpression indicates potential responsiveness to targeted therapies like trastuzumab or lapatinib. Genetic testing can identify patients who are likely to benefit from these targeted therapies, leading to improved treatment outcomes.

4. Optimizing Drug Dosing:
   - Genetic variations can influence drug metabolism and clearance rates, impacting drug efficacy and toxicity. Pharmacogenomic testing can identify patients with genetic variations in drug-metabolizing enzymes or transporters, such as cytochrome P450 enzymes or UGT1A1, allowing for tailored drug dosing strategies. This optimization minimizes the risk of adverse drug reactions and enhances treatment outcomes.

5. Overcoming Drug Resistance:

   • Pharmacogenomics can help identify genetic mechanisms underlying drug resistance in cancer. Resistance to chemotherapy drugs can be caused by specific genetic alterations, such as mutations in drug target genes or DNA repair genes.

   By understanding these genetic mechanisms, clinicians can develop alternative treatment strategies to overcome drug resistance and improve patient outcomes.

6. Clinical Trial Design and Development:

   • Pharmacogenomic information is increasingly integrated into clinical trial design and development. Genetic biomarkers are used to stratify patient populations, allowing for more precise evaluation of treatment efficacy and toxicity. This approach helps identify subpopulations that may benefit the most from specific therapies, leading to more efficient clinical trial outcomes.

7. Future Perspectives:

   • As our understanding of cancer genomics and pharmacogenomics expands, the field of personalized cancer treatment continues to evolve. Emerging technologies, such as liquid biopsies and next-generation sequencing, offer new opportunities for comprehensive profiling of tumors and identification of actionable genetic alterations.

These advancements hold promise for further improving personalized cancer treatment strategies. Pharmacogenomics in oncology holds immense potential for optimizing cancer treatment and improving patient outcomes. By incorporating genetic information into treatment decision-making, clinicians can tailor therapies to individual patients, maximizing efficacy while minimizing toxicity. Continued research and technological advancements in this field are expected to drive further advancements in personalized cancer treatment.

Genetic markers and variations influencing chemotherapy response and toxicity

Genetic markers and variations can significantly influence an individual's response to chemotherapy and their susceptibility to treatment-related toxicity. Understanding these genetic factors is essential for personalized cancer treatment. Here are some key genetic markers and variations that impact chemotherapy response and toxicity:

1. Drug Metabolizing Enzymes:

    - Cytochrome P450 (CYP) enzymes play a vital role in the metabolism of many chemotherapy drugs. Genetic variations in genes encoding these enzymes, such as CYP2D6, CYP2C9, and CYP3A4, can affect the rate at which drugs are metabolized. Variations in these genes may result in altered drug levels, affecting both drug efficacy and toxicity.

2. Drug Transporters:

   • ATP-binding cassette (ABC) transporters, such as ABCB1 (P-glycoprotein) and ABCC2 (MRP2), are involved in the transport of chemotherapy drugs across cell membranes. Genetic variations in these transporter genes can impact drug uptake and efflux, influencing drug levels within cells and altering treatment response and toxicity.

3. DNA Repair Genes:

   • Genetic variations in DNA repair genes can affect an individual's ability to repair chemotherapy-induced DNA damage. For example, variations in BRCA1 and BRCA2 genes have been associated with increased sensitivity to DNA-damaging agents like platinum-based drugs. Conversely, alterations in other DNA repair genes, such as XRCC1 and ERCC1, may contribute to resistance to certain chemotherapy drugs.

4. Drug Target Genes:

   • Genetic variations in genes encoding drug targets can influence drug response. For instance, variations in the epidermal growth factor receptor (EGFR) gene have been associated with response to EGFR inhibitors like gefitinib or erlotinib in lung cancer. Similarly, variations in the HER2 gene impact the response to HER2-targeted therapies like trastuzumab in breast cancer.

5. TP53 Tumor Suppressor Gene:

   - TP53 is a well-known tumor suppressor gene involved in regulating cell cycle progression and DNA repair. Mutations in TP53 are frequently observed in various cancers and can affect treatment outcomes. Patients with TP53 mutations may exhibit altered responses to chemotherapy and may require alternative treatment strategies.

6. Glutathione-S-transferase (GST) Genes:

   - Glutathione-S-transferase enzymes are involved in detoxifying reactive drug metabolites. Variations in GST genes, such as GSTM1 and GSTT1, have been associated with differences in drug metabolism and susceptibility to chemotherapy-induced toxicity. Some genetic variations may result in reduced detoxification capacity, leading to increased drug toxicity.

It is important to note that the influence of these genetic markers and variations on chemotherapy response and toxicity can vary depending on the specific chemotherapy drugs used and the type of cancer. Therefore, comprehensive genetic testing and interpretation, along with clinical considerations, are crucial for guiding treatment decisions and optimizing personalized chemotherapy regimens. Pharmacogenomic testing plays a crucial role in selecting targeted therapies for cancer treatment.

By analyzing specific genetic markers, clinicians can identify patients who are likely to benefit from targeted therapies, allowing for a more personalized and effective approach. Here are some key aspects of pharmacogenomic testing for selecting targeted therapies in cancer treatment:

1. Predictive Biomarkers:

    - Pharmacogenomic testing helps identify predictive biomarkers that indicate a patient's likelihood of responding to a specific targeted therapy. These biomarkers can be genetic alterations, such as mutations, amplifications, or rearrangements in specific genes or pathways.

        Testing for these biomarkers enables clinicians to tailor treatment choices based on the individual's genomic profile.

2. HER2 Testing in Breast Cancer:

    - Human epidermal growth factor receptor 2 (HER2) is a biomarker used in breast cancer to identify patients who are likely to benefit from HER2-targeted therapies, such as trastuzumab. HER2 testing, typically performed using immunohistochemistry (IHC) or fluorescence in situ hybridization (FISH), helps determine the eligibility of patients for targeted treatment. Positive HER2 status indicates a higher likelihood of response to HER2-targeted therapies.

3. BRAF Mutation Testing in Melanoma:

- BRAF is a gene that is frequently mutated in melanoma. Testing for BRAF mutations, such as the V600E mutation, helps identify patients who may benefit from BRAF inhibitors like vemurafenib or dabrafenib.

  BRAF mutation status guides treatment decisions and can significantly impact treatment response and patient outcomes.

4. EGFR Testing in Lung Cancer:

- Epidermal growth factor receptor (EGFR) mutation testing is essential in non-small cell lung cancer (NSCLC) to guide the selection of EGFR tyrosine kinase inhibitors (TKIs) such as erlotinib or gefitinib. Identification of activating EGFR mutations helps identify patients who are more likely to respond to EGFR TKIs, while those with EGFR resistance mutations may require alternative treatment strategies.

5. ALK and ROS1 Testing in Lung Cancer:

- Testing for rearrangements in the anaplastic lymphoma kinase (ALK) and ROS1 genes is crucial in NSCLC. Detection of ALK or ROS1 rearrangements helps identify patients eligible for targeted therapies, such as crizotinib or entrectinib. Targeting these specific gene rearrangements has shown significant clinical benefits in terms of response rates and progression-free survival.

6. MSI and dMMR Testing in Colorectal Cancer:

- Microsatellite instability (MSI) and mismatch repair deficiency (dMMR) testing are performed in colorectal cancer to identify patients who may benefit from immune checkpoint inhibitors, such as pembrolizumab. Testing for MSI or dMMR status helps identify tumors with high immunogenicity, indicating a potential response to immunotherapy.

Pharmacogenomic testing for selecting targeted therapies in cancer treatment is an evolving field. As our understanding of cancer genomics advances, new biomarkers and targeted therapies are continuously being discovered. Incorporating pharmacogenomic testing into clinical practice allows for personalized treatment decisions, maximizing the likelihood of response to targeted therapies and improving patient outcomes.

Here are some case studies highlighting the use of pharmacogenomics in oncology:
Case Study 1: HER2-Positive Breast Cancer and Trastuzumab
In this case study, a 45-year-old female patient is diagnosed with HER2-positive breast cancer. HER2 testing reveals overexpression of the HER2 gene, indicating a higher likelihood of response to HER2-targeted therapies. Based on this finding, the patient receives trastuzumab, a monoclonal antibody that specifically targets the HER2 receptor.

Outcome: The patient shows a significant response to trastuzumab, with a reduction in tumor size and improved progression-free survival. The targeted therapy specifically inhibits HER2 signaling pathways, leading to tumor regression, and improved overall survival rates in HER2-positive breast cancer patients.

Case Study 2: EGFR-Mutated Lung Cancer and EGFR Tyrosine Kinase Inhibitors

A 58-year-old male patient is diagnosed with non-small cell lung cancer (NSCLC). Molecular profiling of the tumor reveals the presence of an EGFR activating mutation (exon 19 deletion). This genetic alteration indicates a higher likelihood of response to EGFR tyrosine kinase inhibitors (TKIs).

Outcome: The patient is treated with an EGFR TKI, such as erlotinib or gefitinib. As a result, the patient experiences a significant reduction in tumor size, improved quality of life, and prolonged progression-free survival. Targeting the specific EGFR mutation helps inhibit aberrant signaling pathways, leading to tumor regression and improved outcomes in EGFR-mutated NSCLC.

Case Study 3: BRAF-Mutated Melanoma and BRAF Inhibitors

A 50-year-old male patient presents with advanced melanoma. Genetic testing reveals the presence of a BRAF V600E mutation, indicating a potential response to BRAF inhibitors. The patient is started on vemurafenib, a BRAF inhibitor.

Outcome: The patient demonstrates a remarkable response to vemurafenib, with a significant reduction in tumor size and improved overall survival.

Targeting the specific BRAF mutation inhibits aberrant signaling in melanoma cells, leading to tumor regression and improved outcomes in BRAF-mutated melanoma.

These case studies highlight the clinical utility of pharmacogenomics in oncology. By identifying specific genetic alterations, such as HER2 overexpression, EGFR mutations, or BRAF mutations, clinicians can select targeted therapies that have a higher likelihood of success. Pharmacogenomic testing allows for a more personalized and precise approach to cancer treatment, leading to improved treatment outcomes and better patient care.

For example, the drug vemurafenib was developed to treat melanoma patients with a specific mutation in the BRAF gene, which is found in about 50% of melanomas. Similarly, the drug crizotinib targets a specific gene fusion in lung cancer, and olaparib is used to treat ovarian cancer patients with a BRCA mutation.

Pharmacogenomics can also be used to predict a patient's response to chemotherapy, allowing oncologists to tailor the treatment plan to maximize effectiveness while minimizing toxicity. For example, a study published in the New England Journal of Medicine found that breast cancer patients with a specific genetic variant had a significantly higher response rate to the chemotherapy drug paclitaxel than patients without the variant.

Another example of the use of pharmacogenomics in oncology is in the identification of patients who are at increased risk of developing certain cancers based on their genetic profile.

For example, individuals with mutations in the BRCA1 or BRCA2 genes are at increased risk of developing breast and ovarian cancer and may choose to undergo preventive measures such as prophylactic surgery or increased surveillance.

The use of pharmacogenomics in oncology holds great promise for improving treatment outcomes and reducing toxicity in cancer patients. However, more research is needed to fully realize the potential of this approach, and to ensure that it is implemented in an ethical and equitable manner.

Chapter 9: Pharmacogenomics in Gastroenterology and Hepatology

Genetic factors can influence the response to medications used in the treatment of gastrointestinal disorders, including inflammatory bowel disease (IBD) and gastroesophageal reflux disease (GERD). Here are some key genetic considerations:

1. Inflammatory Bowel Disease (IBD): a. Thiopurine Methyltransferase (TPMT) Genotype: TPMT is an enzyme involved in the metabolism of thiopurine medications, such as azathioprine and mercaptopurine, commonly used in the treatment of IBD. Genetic variations in the TPMT gene can lead to reduced enzyme activity, resulting in increased drug toxicity and a higher risk of myelosuppression. Genetic testing for TPMT variants can help identify individuals who are at higher risk for adverse reactions and guide dosing adjustments.

   b. NOD2/CARD15 Genotype: Variations in the NOD2 gene, also known as the CARD15 gene, have been associated with an increased risk of developing Crohn's disease, a type of IBD. Additionally, certain NOD2 variants may influence treatment response to anti-tumor necrosis factor (TNF) agents, such as infliximab and adalimumab. Pharmacogenomic testing for NOD2 variants can assist in personalized treatment decisions for patients with Crohn's disease.

2. Gastroesophageal Reflux Disease (GERD): a. CYP2C19 Genotype: The CYP2C19 gene encodes an enzyme involved in the metabolism of proton pump inhibitors (PPIs), such as omeprazole and lansoprazole, commonly prescribed for GERD. Genetic variations in CYP2C19 can lead to differences in drug metabolism and plasma concentrations. Poor metabolizers may require lower doses of PPIs, while ultrarapid metabolizers may need higher doses for effective symptom control. Pharmacogenomic testing for CYP2C19 variants can guide individualized dosing strategies for PPIs. b. OXTR Genotype: Variations in the oxytocin receptor gene (OXTR) have been associated with differences in the response to treatments targeting esophageal motility and reflux symptoms. Genetic testing for OXTR variants may help identify individuals who are more likely to respond to certain medications, such as baclofen or nitrates.

It's important to note that while genetic factors can provide valuable insights, they should be considered in conjunction with other clinical factors and guidelines when making treatment decisions.

Pharmacogenomic testing can assist clinicians in personalized prescribing and optimizing treatment outcomes, but it should be integrated with comprehensive clinical assessments and ongoing monitoring of patients' responses to medication. Additionally, genetic testing for gastrointestinal disorders is not yet as well-established as in some other areas of medicine, so its use and interpretation may vary depending on the specific clinical context.

Pharmacogenomics can play a role in the treatment of liver diseases, including hepatitis C and non-alcoholic fatty liver disease (NAFLD). Here are some key considerations for the pharmacogenomics of drugs used in the treatment of liver diseases:

1. Hepatitis C: a. Direct-Acting Antivirals (DAAs): DAAs, such as sofosbuvir, ledipasvir, and daclatasvir, are highly effective in treating hepatitis C virus (HCV) infection. Genetic variations in the IL28B gene, specifically the IL28B genotype (rs12979860), have been found to influence treatment response rates. Individuals with specific IL28B genotypes, such as CC genotype, have shown higher response rates to DAAs. Pharmacogenomic testing for IL28B genotypes can help predict treatment response and guide treatment decisions. b. Ribavirin: Ribavirin is sometimes used in combination with DAAs for the treatment of hepatitis C. Genetic variations in the inosine triphosphatase (ITPA) gene have been associated with ribavirin-induced hemolytic anemia. Testing for ITPA variants can identify individuals at higher risk of developing anemia and help guide ribavirin dosing or alternative treatment strategies.

2. Non-alcoholic Fatty Liver Disease (NAFLD): a. Vitamin E: Vitamin E has been used as a therapeutic option for non-alcoholic steatohepatitis (NASH), a progressive form of NAFLD.

Genetic variations in the patatin-like phospholipase domain-containing 3 (PNPLA3) gene have been associated with NAFLD/NASH susceptibility and response to treatment with vitamin E. Testing for PNPLA3 variants can help stratify patients based on their genetic risk and guide treatment decisions. b. Pioglitazone: Pioglitazone, a medication commonly used to treat type 2 diabetes, has shown some benefit in the treatment of NASH. Genetic variations in the peroxisome proliferator-activated receptor gamma (PPARG) gene have been associated with response to pioglitazone in NASH patients. Pharmacogenomic testing for PPARG variants can help identify individuals who may be more likely to respond to pioglitazone therapy.

It's important to note that while pharmacogenomic testing can provide valuable information, its use in the context of liver diseases is still evolving.

The available evidence and clinical guidelines for pharmacogenomic testing in liver diseases may vary, and testing may be more established for certain medications and genetic markers compared to others. Additionally, the influence of genetic factors may differ among different populations. Therefore, it is essential to consider the specific clinical context, individual patient characteristics, and available evidence when integrating pharmacogenomic information into the treatment of liver diseases.

Pharmacogenomics plays a significant role in optimizing therapy and reducing adverse events in the fields of gastroenterology and hepatology. Here are some key aspects of how pharmacogenomics can be applied:

1. Personalized Medication Selection: Pharmacogenomic testing can help identify genetic variations that impact drug metabolism, efficacy, and safety. This information enables clinicians to choose medications that are more likely to be effective and well-tolerated by individual patients. For example, genetic testing can determine a patient's metabolizer status for drugs such as thiopurines (used in inflammatory bowel disease) or proton pump inhibitors (used in gastroesophageal reflux disease). This knowledge guides medication selection and appropriate dosing adjustments to optimize therapy outcomes.

2. Prediction of Treatment Response: Genetic variations can influence an individual's response to specific medications used in gastroenterology and hepatology. Pharmacogenomic testing can help predict treatment response, enabling clinicians to select the most effective medication for each patient. For example, in hepatitis C treatment, testing for the IL28B genotype can identify patients with a higher likelihood of responding to direct-acting antiviral therapy.

3. Identification of Drug-Related Adverse Events: Some adverse drug reactions are associated with specific genetic variations. Pharmacogenomic testing can identify patients at increased risk of adverse events, enabling clinicians to choose alternative medications or adjust dosages accordingly.

For example, testing for HLA-B*57:01 genotype can help identify individuals at high risk of developing severe hypersensitivity reactions to abacavir, a medication used in HIV treatment.

4. Dosing Optimization: Genetic factors can impact drug metabolism and clearance, leading to variations in drug concentrations in the body. Pharmacogenomic testing can provide insights into optimal dosing strategies for medications in gastroenterology and hepatology. For instance, testing for CYP2C19 genetic variations can guide dosing adjustments for proton pump inhibitors to achieve adequate acid suppression.

5. Treatment of Hepatitis B: Pharmacogenomics can assist in the management of chronic hepatitis B by identifying genetic markers associated with drug response. For example, genetic variations in the UDP-glucuronosyltransferase 1A1 (UGT1A1) gene influence the metabolism of entecavir, a commonly used antiviral medication. Pharmacogenomic testing can help determine the appropriate dosage for individuals with specific UGT1A1 genotypes.

It's important to note that while pharmacogenomic testing can provide valuable information, it should be integrated into comprehensive clinical assessments and guidelines. The field of pharmacogenomics is continually evolving, and more research is needed to establish evidence-based guidelines for specific medications and genetic markers in gastroenterology and hepatology.

Collaboration between gastroenterologists, hepatologists, and clinical pharmacologists is crucial to effectively implement pharmacogenomic information into clinical practice and optimize therapy while reducing adverse events.

Here are a few case studies illustrating the application of pharmacogenomics in gastroenterology and hepatology:

1. Case Study: Thiopurine Pharmacogenomics in Inflammatory Bowel Disease: A case report published in Clinical Gastroenterology and Hepatology in 2019 described a patient with inflammatory bowel disease (IBD) who experienced severe myelosuppression following treatment with thiopurine medications (azathioprine). Pharmacogenomic testing was performed to identify genetic variations in the thiopurine methyltransferase (TPMT) gene. The patient was found to have a TPMT variant associated with reduced enzyme activity. Based on the test results, the patient's thiopurine dose was adjusted to prevent further myelosuppression, resulting in improved tolerability and treatment response.

2. Case Study: Genetic Testing for Anti-TNF Therapy in Crohn's Disease: In a case study published in Digestive Diseases and Sciences in 2014, a patient with Crohn's disease underwent pharmacogenomic testing to guide the selection of anti-tumor necrosis factor (TNF) therapy.

The patient had previously failed multiple anti-TNF medications. Genetic testing was performed to identify variations in the NOD2/CARD15 gene associated with Crohn's disease susceptibility and response to anti-TNF therapy. The results indicated the presence of a variant associated with a reduced likelihood of responding to anti-TNF therapy. Based on the test results, the patient was switched to a different medication with a different mechanism of action, resulting in significant improvement in symptoms and disease remission.

3. Case Study: Pharmacogenomics of Proton Pump Inhibitors in Gastroesophageal Reflux Disease: A case report published in the Journal of Clinical Gastroenterology in 2016 highlighted the role of pharmacogenomics in optimizing proton pump inhibitor (PPI) therapy for gastroesophageal reflux disease (GERD). The patient experienced suboptimal response to standard PPI dosing. Pharmacogenomic testing was performed to assess variations in the CYP2C19 gene, which is involved in PPI metabolism.

   The patient was found to be a poor metabolizer due to a specific CYP2C19 variant, resulting in reduced drug efficacy. Adjustments were made to the PPI dosage based on the test results, leading to improved symptom control and resolution of GERD-related complications.

These case studies demonstrate how pharmacogenomic testing can guide medication selection, dosing adjustments, and treatment response in gastroenterology and hepatology. By considering an individual's genetic variations, clinicians can personalize treatment strategies, enhance medication efficacy, and minimize the risk of adverse events. However, it's important to note that these case studies represent specific scenarios, and pharmacogenomic testing recommendations may vary based on individual patient characteristics, clinical guidelines, and available testing resources.

Chapter 10: Ethical and Social Issues

As with any emerging field of science and technology, pharmacogenomics raises several ethical and social concerns that must be considered. Some of the key ethical considerations in pharmacogenomics include issues of informed consent, privacy and confidentiality, and the potential for discrimination.

One of the main ethical concerns in pharmacogenomics is the potential for discrimination based on genetic information. Discrimination can take many forms, including denial of insurance coverage, employment discrimination, or even social stigma. For example, genetic testing for the BRCA1 and BRCA2 genes, which are associated with an increased risk of breast and ovarian cancer, has raised concerns about discrimination against individuals who test positive for these genes.

Another ethical concern in pharmacogenomics is the issue of informed consent. Patients must be fully informed about the nature of the test, the potential risks and benefits, and the implications of the results before they agree to undergo testing. Additionally, patients must have the right to refuse testing if they so choose.

Privacy and confidentiality are also important ethical considerations in pharmacogenomics. Genetic information is highly personal and sensitive, and patients have the right to expect that their information will be kept confidential and protected from unauthorized access or disclosure. However, there is always the risk of breaches in data security and privacy, which can lead to discrimination and other negative consequences.

The Genetic Information Nondiscrimination Act (GINA) is a federal law in the United States that prohibits employers and health insurers from using an individual's genetic information to discriminate against them. It was signed into law in 2008 and is enforced by the Equal Employment Opportunity Commission (EEOC) and the Department of Health and Human Services (HHS). GINA defines genetic information broadly, including an individual's own genetic tests, family members' genetic tests, and family medical history.

Under GINA, employers cannot use genetic information in employment decisions, and health insurers cannot use it to deny coverage, raise premiums, or impose any adverse treatment.

GINA also prohibits retaliation against individuals who file complaints or participate in investigations related to genetic discrimination. In the context of pharmacogenomics, GINA is critical in protecting individuals' genetic information and ensuring that they are not discriminated against in employment or health insurance.

As pharmacogenomics testing becomes more prevalent, GINA provides important protections to allow individuals to undergo testing without fear of negative consequences. However, GINA has some limitations, such as not covering life insurance, long-term care insurance, or disability insurance, leaving individuals vulnerable to discrimination in these areas. Additionally, GINA does not extend protection to discrimination in other areas of life, such as education or housing.

Despite these limitations, GINA represents a significant step forward in protecting the rights of individuals with genetic conditions or predispositions. As pharmacogenomics continues to advance and become more widely used, it is important to ensure that GINA and other laws and regulations keep up with these developments to prevent unfair discrimination based on genetic information.

There are also social implications of pharmacogenomics to consider. Social implications of pharmacogenomics include issues related to access to testing and treatment. As with many new medical technologies, pharmacogenomics testing may be more readily available to those who can afford it, leading to disparities in access to care. Additionally, the development of targeted medications based on genetic profiles may lead to higher costs, which could limit access to treatment for some patients.

The availability of testing and treatment may be limited to certain populations, leading to disparities in access to care. Additionally, targeted medications based on genetic profiles may be more expensive, which could limit access to treatment for some patients.

Despite these concerns, pharmacogenomics has the potential to improve outcomes and reduce adverse drug reactions by tailoring medication therapy to a patient's unique genetic profile. For example, genetic testing for HLA-B*5701 can help identify patients at risk for hypersensitivity reactions to the HIV drug abacavir, allowing clinicians to prescribe an alternative medication.

Pharmacogenomics research may help us better understand the underlying causes of disease and identify new targets for drug development. It is important to carefully consider the ethical and social implications of pharmacogenomics as we continue to develop and implement these technologies. Policies and regulations must be put in place to ensure that genetic information is used responsibly and that patients are protected from discrimination and other negative consequences.

Chapter 11: Current and Future Directions

Pharmacogenomics is a rapidly evolving field with many promising future applications. Here are some of the current research areas and potential future directions for pharmacogenomics:

1. Precision medicine: The goal of pharmacogenomics is to enable precision medicine, where treatment is tailored to the unique genetic profile of each patient. Advances in pharmacogenomics may lead to more personalized treatment approaches, better outcomes, and fewer adverse drug reactions.

2. Gene editing: Gene editing techniques like CRISPR-Cas9 may one day be used to correct genetic variations that affect drug response. While this is still largely theoretical, it has the potential to revolutionize pharmacogenomics by allowing us to directly target and modify the genetic variants that contribute to disease.

3. Pharmacogenomics in clinical trials: Incorporating pharmacogenomic testing into clinical trials could help identify which patients are most likely to benefit from a particular treatment, improving trial efficiency and reducing costs.

4. Biomarker discovery: Pharmacogenomics research may lead to the discovery of new biomarkers that can be used to identify patients who are at risk for adverse drug reactions or who are most likely to benefit from a particular treatment.

5. Population-level studies: Large-scale studies of genetic variation and drug response across populations could help us better understand the genetic and environmental factors that contribute to variability in drug response. This information could be used to develop more effective treatment approaches and to improve drug safety.

6. Artificial intelligence and machine learning: Advances in artificial intelligence and machine learning may enable us to better analyze and interpret large-scale pharmacogenomic data sets, leading to more accurate predictions of drug response and more personalized treatment recommendations.

Future direction

Pharmacogenomics is an evolving field that holds great promise for improving personalized medicine and optimizing drug therapy. Some potential future directions for pharmacogenomics include:

1. Integration into routine clinical practice: As pharmacogenomic testing becomes more accessible and cost-effective, it is likely to become more widely adopted in routine clinical practice. This could lead to improved patient outcomes and reduced healthcare costs by helping doctors identify the most effective medications and dosages for each patient.

2. Development of new drugs: Pharmacogenomic research may help identify new drug targets and pathways that can be exploited for the development of

novel therapeutics. By understanding the genetic basis of disease, researchers may be able to develop drugs that are more targeted and effective, with fewer side effects.

3. Expansion of pharmacogenomic testing to non-drug therapies: While pharmacogenomics has traditionally focused on drug therapy, it may also have applications in non-drug therapies such as gene therapy or immunotherapy. By understanding how genetic variations affect the response to these therapies, researchers may be able to improve their efficacy and reduce side effects.

4. Integration with other technologies: As technology continues to advance, pharmacogenomics may be integrated with other technologies such as artificial intelligence or wearable devices to provide real-time monitoring of drug response and optimize treatment on an individual basis.

5. Public health initiatives: Pharmacogenomics may also have applications in public health initiatives such as population screening for genetic variations associated with drug response. By identifying individuals who are at risk for adverse drug reactions, public health initiatives may be able to reduce healthcare costs and improve overall population health.

Overall, pharmacogenomics has the potential to revolutionize the field of medicine by providing personalized and effective treatments based on an individual's unique genetic profile.

As research in this field continues to advance, we can expect to see many exciting new developments in the years to come.

Nutrigenomics: Unveiling the Interplay Between Genetics and Nutrition

In the realm of scientific discovery, few fields have captured the imagination and potential of personalized healthcare like nutrigenomics. This groundbreaking discipline delves into the intricate relationship between genetics and nutrition, shedding light on how our unique genetic makeup influences our response to different foods and dietary components. Nutrigenomics has revolutionized our understanding of how individualized dietary interventions can optimize health outcomes and prevent chronic diseases.

1. Genetics and Nutrition Unveiled

At the heart of nutrigenomics lies the realization that our genes hold the key to how our bodies interact with the foods we consume. Every individual inherits a unique genetic blueprint that governs the synthesis and function of proteins, enzymes, and receptors involved in digestion, metabolism, and nutrient utilization. The interactions between these genetic factors and dietary components form the foundation of nutrigenomics.

For instance, the FTO gene has been linked to obesity risk. Individuals carrying certain variants of this gene might be more susceptible to weight gain when consuming diets high in saturated fats. On the other hand, those with a specific variant of the APOE gene might have a heightened sensitivity to dietary cholesterol, impacting their cardiovascular health.

2. The Role of Epigenetics

Nutrigenomics also delves into the realm of epigenetics, where environmental factors, including diet, can modify the expression of genes without altering the underlying DNA sequence. Epigenetic changes have the potential to be inherited, allowing dietary habits to influence not only an individual's health but also that of future generations.

Methylation, a common epigenetic modification, is influenced by nutrients like folate and B vitamins. These nutrients play a pivotal role in regulating gene expression, with deficiencies potentially leading to increased disease susceptibility. For instance, studies have shown that maternal diets rich in methyl donors can influence the risk of obesity and metabolic disorders in offspring.

3. Personalized Nutrition for Optimal Health

One of the most exciting aspects of nutrigenomics is its ability to guide personalized dietary recommendations. By analyzing an individual's genetic profile, healthcare professionals can tailor dietary plans that align with their genetic predispositions. This approach has the potential to enhance nutrient absorption, reduce disease risk, and optimize overall health outcomes.

For instance, a person with a genetic tendency towards poor vitamin D metabolism might require higher levels of supplementation to maintain optimal bone health. Another example involves caffeine metabolism, where genetic variations impact how quickly caffeine is processed. This insight can guide individuals on their coffee consumption to avoid potential negative effects.

Conclusion:

Nutrigenomics represents a monumental leap forward in the quest for personalized healthcare. By decoding the intricate interplay between genetics and nutrition, this field has the power to transform the way we approach diet and health. The examples discussed here merely scratch the surface of the vast potential that nutrigenomics holds, offering a glimpse into a future where diets are tailored to individual genetic profiles, ushering in an era of truly personalized nutrition.

Chapter 12: Resources for Pharmacogenomics and Conclusion

There are many resources available for learning more about pharmacogenomics, including websites, organizations, and other educational materials. Here are some examples:

1. Pharmacogenomics Knowledgebase (PharmGKB): A comprehensive online resource that provides information about how genetic variations affect drug response, as well as guidance on how to use this information in clinical practice. https://www.pharmgkb.org/

2. National Human Genome Research Institute: The NHGRI is a division of the National Institutes of Health that supports research into the genetic basis of disease, including pharmacogenomics. Their website provides a wealth of information about genetics and genomics, including educational resources for healthcare providers and patients. https://www.genome.gov/

3. Clinical Pharmacogenetics Implementation Consortium (CPIC): A consortium of experts in pharmacogenomics that provides guidelines for how to use genetic information to inform medication therapy. Their website provides a searchable database of medication-gene pairs and corresponding dosing recommendations based on genotype. https://cpicpgx.org/

4. U.S. Food and Drug Administration (FDA): The FDA regulates the safety and efficacy of drugs and medical devices in the U.S. and has a growing interest in pharmacogenomics. Their website provides information about how the agency is incorporating genetic information into drug development and regulation. https://www.fda.gov/

5. American Society of Clinical Pharmacology and Therapeutics (ASCPT): ASCPT is a professional society for pharmacologists and other healthcare professionals who are interested in clinical pharmacology and therapeutics. Their website provides educational resources and training opportunities for members. https://www.ascpt.org/

6. International Conference on Pharmacoepigenomics: A biennial conference that brings together researchers, clinicians, and other experts in pharmacogenomics and epigenomics to discuss the latest advances in the field. https://pharmacoepigenomics.org/

These are just a few examples of the many resources available for learning more about pharmacogenomics. Healthcare providers, patients, and researchers alike can benefit from exploring these and other resources to stay up to date on the latest developments in this exciting field.

Pharmacogenomics is a rapidly evolving field that has the potential to revolutionize medicine by tailoring treatment to a patient's unique genetic profile. By analyzing a patient's DNA, pharmacogenomics can identify genetic variations that may affect their response to medications, allowing doctors to optimize therapy and improve patient outcomes. This approach to personalized medicine has already had a significant impact in several areas of healthcare, including oncology, cardiology, and psychiatry.

One of the key benefits of pharmacogenomics is its ability to reduce the risk of adverse drug reactions, which are a significant cause of morbidity and mortality. By identifying patients who are at increased risk of adverse reactions, pharmacogenomics can help doctors choose the most appropriate medication and dosage, reducing the risk of harm. Additionally, pharmacogenomics can help identify patients who may not respond to a particular medication, allowing doctors to choose an alternative therapy that is more likely to be effective.

Pharmacogenomics also has the potential to improve the efficiency of clinical trials and drug development. By stratifying patients based on their genetic profiles, clinical trials can be designed to include only those patients who are most likely to respond to the medication being tested. This can reduce the number of patients needed for the trial, making the process faster and more cost-effective.

Overall, pharmacogenomics represents a major shift in the way we approach healthcare, moving away from a one-size-fits-all approach to personalized medicine that is tailored to the individual.

As research in this field continues to expand, we can expect to see even more applications of pharmacogenomics in clinical practice, leading to better outcomes for patients and a more efficient healthcare system. pharmacogenomics represents an exciting and rapidly growing field with the potential to transform the way we practice medicine and improve patient outcomes. It is important that we continue to invest in research and education in this area to realize the full potential of this important field.

References

1. Evans WE, Relling MV. Pharmacogenomics: translating functional genomics into rational therapeutics. Science. 1999;286(5439):487-491.

2. Johnson JA. Pharmacogenetics in clinical practice: how far have we come and where are we going? Pharmacogenomics. 2013;14(7):835-843.

3. Relling MV, Evans WE. Pharmacogenomics in the clinic. Nature. 2015;526(7573):343-350.

4. Holford NH. Clinical pharmacokinetics and pharmacodynamics: concepts and applications. 4th ed. Philadelphia: Lippincott Williams & Wilkins; 2005.

5. Zanger UM, Schwab M. Cytochrome P450 enzymes in drug metabolism: regulation of gene expression, enzyme activities, and impact of genetic variation. Pharmacol Ther. 2013;138(1):103-41.

6. Tuteja S, Haynes K, Piccirillo JF, et al. Genomic knowledge for personalized medicine: the case of clopidogrel. Pharmacogenomics. 2013;14(3):243-251.

7. Yin T, Miyata T. Warfarin dose and the pharmacogenomics of CYP2C9 and VKORC1 - rationale and perspectives. Thromb Res. 2007;120(1):1-10.

8. Kwiatkowski DP. How malaria has affected the human genome and what human genetics can teach us about malaria. Am J Hum Genet. 2005

Nov;77(5):171-92. doi: 10.1086/432519. PMID: 16252235; PMCID: PMC1275616.

9. Feuk L, Carson AR, Scherer SW. Structural variation in the human genome. Nat Rev Genet. 2006 Nov;7(11):85-97. doi: 10.1038/nrg1767. PMID: 17047681.

10. Alkan C, Coe BP, Eichler EE. Genome structural variation discovery and genotyping. Nat Rev Genet. 2011 Mar;12(5):363-76. doi: 10.1038/nrg2958. PMID: 21448239; PMCID: PMC3525150.

11. Clinical Pharmacogenetics Implementation Consortium (CPIC). https://cpicpgx.org/. Accessed May 8, 2023.

12. Crews KR, Hicks JK, Pui CH, Relling MV, Evans WE. Pharmacogenomics and individualized medicine: translating science into practice. Clin Pharmacol Ther. 2012 Sep;92(3):467-75. doi: 10.1038/clpt.2012.96. Epub 2012 Jul 18. PMID: 22810788.

13. Van Driest SL, Shi Y, Bowton EA, Schildcrout JS, Peterson JF, Pulley J, Denny JC, Roden DM. Clinically actionable genotypes among 10,000 patients with preemptive pharmacogenomic testing. Clin Pharmacol Ther. 2014 Oct;96(4):391-8. doi: 10.1038/clpt.2014.132. Epub 2014 Jul 28. PMID: 25069936.

14. O'Donnell PH, Bush A, Spitz J, Danahey K, Saner D, Das S, Cox NJ, Ratain MJ. The 1200 Patients Project: creating a new medical model system for

clinical implementation of pharmacogenomics. Clin Pharmacol Ther. 2012 Sep;92(3):446-9. doi: 10.1038/clpt.2012.119. PMID: 22829168.

15. Swen JJ, Nijenhuis M, de Boer A, et al. Pharmacogenetics: from bench to byte--an update of guidelines. Clin Pharmacol Ther. 2011;89(5):662-673.

16. Weitzel KW, Elsey AR, Langaee TY, Burkley B, Nessl DR, Obeng AO, et al. Clinical pharmacogenetics implementation consortium guidelines for CYP2C9 and HLA-B genotypes and phenytoin dosing. Clin Pharmacol Ther. 2013;93(4):324-327.

17. Haga SB, Mills R, Moaddeb J. Pharmacogenetic testing: perspectives from the Department of Veterans Affairs. Pharmacogenomics. 2013;14(6):611-614.

18. Kitzmiller JP, Daneshjou R, Ratain MJ, et al. Pharmacogenomics of statins: understanding susceptibility to adverse effects. Pharmacogenomics J. 2014;14(2):93-106. doi:10.1038/tpj.2013.2

19. Fabbri, C., Porcelli, S., Serretti, A. (2018). From pharmacogenetics to pharmacogenomics: The way toward the personalization of antidepressant treatment. Canadian Journal of Psychiatry, 63(12), 809-817.

20. Ledermann JA, Harter P, Gourley C, et al. Olaparib maintenance therapy in patients with platinum-sensitive relapsed serous ovarian cancer: a preplanned retrospective analysis of outcomes by BRCA status in a randomized phase 2 trial. Lancet Oncol. 2014;15(8):852-861.

21. Rothstein MA, Epps P. Ethical and legal implications of pharmacogenomics. Nat Rev Genet. 2001;2(3):228-231.

22. Evans JP, Meslin EM. Ethical and social implications of pharmacogenomics. Perspect Biol Med. 2004;47(3):385-398.

23. Joly Y, So D, Osien G, Tremblay M. Ethical and social issues in pharmacogenomics: challenges for public policy. Trends Pharmacol Sci. 2006;27(7):298-301.

24. Dressler LG. Social and ethical implications of pharmacogenomics. Pharmacogenomics. 2004;5(3):293-299.

25. Fullerton SM, Lee SS, Hernandez RD, et al. Ethical issues in the use of whole genome sequencing for public health surveillance: lessons from the human genome diversity panel. PLoS Biol. 2011;9(3):e1001198.

26. Caulfield T, McGuire A. Ethical, legal, and social issues in the translation of genomics into health care. JAMA. 2008;299(11):1355-1359. doi:10.1001/jama.299.11.1355

27. Evans JP, Rothschild BB. Return of results: not that complicated? Genet Med. 2012;14(4):358-360. doi:10.1038/gim.2012.3

28. Ordovas JM. Nutrigenomics and Nutrigenetics. Curr Opin Lipidol. 2004;15(2):101-108.

29. Corella D, Ordovas JM. Nutrigenomics in Cardiovascular Medicine. Circ Cardiovasc Genet. 2009;2(6):637-651.

30. Zeisel SH. Nutrigenomics and Metabolic Disease: Current Status and Implications for Personalized Nutrition. Nutr Rev. 2004;62(11):429-436.

31. Grosse SD, Khoury MJ. What is the clinical utility of genetic testing? Genet Med. 2006;8(7):448-450. doi:10.1097/01.gim.0000237866.52517.2b

32. Green RC, Berg JS, Grody WW, et al. ACMG recommendations for reporting of incidental findings in clinical exome and genome sequencing. Genet Med. 2013;15(7):565-574. doi:10.1038/gim.2013.73

33. Sadee W, Hartmann K, Seweryn M, Pietrzak M, Handelman SK, Rempala GA. Missing heritability of common diseases and treatments outside the protein-coding exome. Hum Genet. 2014 Nov;133(11):1199-215.

34. Denny JC, Rutter JL, Goldstein DB, Philippakis A, Smoller JW, Jenkins G, Dishman E. The "All of Us" Research Program. N Engl J Med. 2019 Jan 3;380(1):e4.

35. Sim SC, Kacevska M, Ingelman-Sundberg M. Pharmacogenomics of drug-metabolizing enzymes: a recent update on clinical implications and endogenous effects. Pharmacogenomics J. 2013 Feb;13(1):1-11.

Made in United States
North Haven, CT
17 April 2024

51442480R00059